Ana Cristina Viera Costa
Maria Cecilia de Sousa Cunha
Maria da Penha Silva do Nascimento

Organisational diagnosis

Ana Cristina Viera Costa
Maria Cecilia de Sousa Cunha
Maria da Penha Silva do Nascimento

Organisational diagnosis

On pig farms in São Luís - ma

ScienciaScripts

Imprint

Cover image: www.ingimage.com

This book is a translation from the original published under ISBN 978-620-6-76153-2.

Publisher:
Sciencia Scripts
is a trademark of
Dodo Books Indian Ocean Ltd. and OmniScriptum S.R.L publishing group

120 High Road, East Finchley, London, N2 9ED, United Kingdom
Str. Armeneasca 28/1, office 1, Chisinau MD-2012, Republic of Moldova, Europe
Managing Directors: Ieva Konstantinova, Victoria Ursu
info@omniscriptum.com

Printed at: see last page
ISBN: 978-620-8-57791-9

Contents

PRESENTATION

This ebook provides students, professionals and producers with the necessary elements to understand and improve all aspects of their pig operation through the management tool that is organisational diagnosis. The authors were guided by two main concerns when preparing the book. Firstly, to introduce students to the SWOT model, which is used to analyse and diagnose the internal and external environment of farms, in a simple and accessible way.

Secondly, it aims to ensure that agricultural professionals and producers can organise their knowledge of pig farming. The content of this ebook translates all the academic and practical knowledge into solutions for the challenges that producers face on a daily basis when dealing with this activity.

Despite its practical nature, this e-book is far from being a "recipe". Throughout its chapters, it attempts to deal with the most diverse theoretical implications surrounding the process of raising pigs.

NOTE ON THE AUTHORS

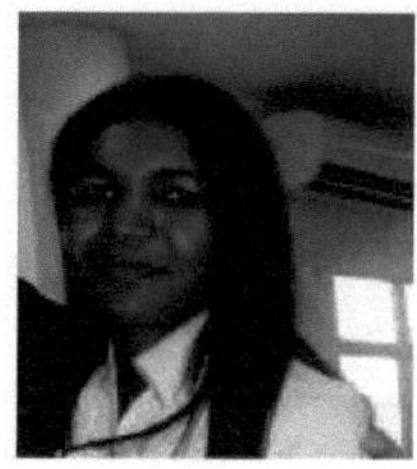

Ana Cristina Vieira Costa Address to access this CV: http://lattes.cnpq.br/8304398061212975 .Last updated on 03/10/2023

ANA CRISTINA VIEIRA COSTA. She has a degree in Zootechnics from the State University of Maranhão (2015) and a degree in Business Administration from the Athens Maranhense College (2013). She is also studying for a degree in Agricultural Sciences at the Federal Institute of Maranhão - IFMA and has a postgraduate degree in Teaching in Higher Education from FUTURA College, a postgraduate degree in Agribusiness from Educaminas College and a postgraduate degree in pig farming and poultry farming, also from Educaminas.

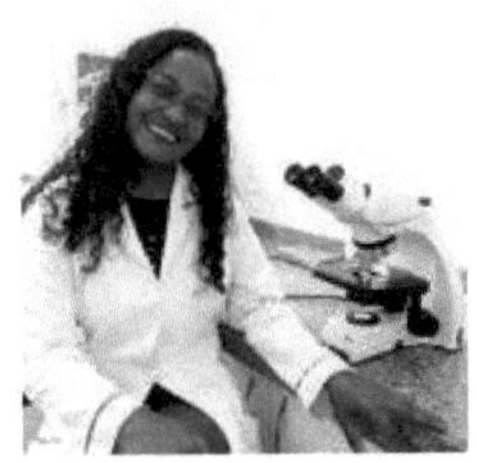

Maria Cecília de Sousa Cunha. Address to access this CV: http://lattes.cnpq.br/9806654948185863ID Lattes: 9806654948185863Last updated on 19/12/2023

MARIA CECILIA DE SOUSA CUNHA. Special PhD student in Animal Defence (State University of Maranhão) (Current), Higher Level Technical Fellow at the Food and Water Quality and Control Laboratory (UEMA) (Current). Master's degree in Animal Science in the area of Preventive Veterinary Medicine/Animal Pathogenesis (UEMA) (2015), Specialisation in Food Health Surveillance (2012), On-site tutor for the Food Technician course at Rede e-Tec Brasil (2013), Head of the UV office in Anajatuba (INAGRO) (2017) and has a degree in Veterinary Medicine from the State University of Maranhão (UEMA) (2010), monitors General Microbiology, Veterinary Microbiology, Microbiology of Animal Products and also small animal husbandry (goats and pigs). She has experience in the field of Veterinary Medicine, with an emphasis on Food and Water Quality Control and Small Animal Veterinary Clinic (dog and cat). (Text provided by the author)

"To have a successful business, someone, sometime, had to take a brave step."

Peter Druck

SUMMARY

The general aim of this study was to carry out an organisational diagnosis of pig farms in the municipality of São Luís - MA. Primary and secondary data were used to carry out this work. To obtain primary data, a questionnaire was administered to fifteen pig producers. As part of the methodology, the SWOT model was used to analyse and diagnose the internal and external environment of the properties analysed. The results showed that all the properties use less than their production capacity, that 93.3% of them have other agricultural activities, that 86.7% of the producers don't control their costs and that 66.7% of the producers don't receive technical assistance. Production is commercialised mainly through live animals, which means that producers are paid less, and 73.3% of producers have no health inspection records, so both the rearing and slaughtering of animals takes place in a clandestine manner.

Keywords: Analysis. Diagnosis. Swot. Rural property.

1 INTRODUCTION

Nowadays, with the strong influences of the external environment such as the opening up of markets, technological advances, the speed of information, new consumer needs and fierce competition, it is necessary for rural producers not only to produce, but also to know what, how and when to produce.

From this perspective, rural producers will have to implement a management approach that changes their attitude and mentality, as their attitudes and behaviour are fundamental in determining the transition from a traditional production system to a rural company that operates strategically. According to Chiavenato (2007), there are countless ways to manage a business, but when looking for models that facilitate the learning of the organisation's managers, with a view to success and obtaining long-term results, it is necessary to understand the decision-making process in search of the organisation's desired performance. According to Chiavenato (2010) in the long term, strategic management increases the company's chances of success in its business, so the agents responsible for decision-making in companies must define functional and coherent plans. In this context, the concern with business strategy and efficiency in operations management in all organisations stands out, in this case as proposed in the study, especially in rural organisations and, more specifically, in those whose main activity is pig farming. For this reason, the need to observe the existence of efficient management mechanisms through business diagnostics is emphasised.

The subject of this work arose from contact with the reality of rural properties, during practical classes in the Zootechnics course, where it became clear that the lack of control of production costs and strategic information for producers to make decisions in favour of their business are common and recurring problems. Associated with this, this subject is dealt with sparsely in the literature, and the relevance of the study is emphasised due to the lack of research on this subject in the context of agricultural activities. The aim was therefore to carry out an organisational diagnosis of pig farms in the municipality of São Luis.

It is known that a strategy represents the alternatives that define the paths that lead to the desired objective. On the other hand, strategy must be related to the organisation's desired performance. This gave rise to the question that guided this research: how can strategy and performance be linked in a rural property environment? There are many ways of managing a business, but when looking for models that make it easier for the organisation's managers to learn, with a view to success and achieving long-term results, it is necessary to understand the decision-making process in pursuit of the organisation's desired performance.

1.1 Objectives

1.1.1 General Objective

To carry out an organisational diagnosis of pig farms in the municipality of São Luis - MA.

1.1.2 Specific objectives

a) Identify the current situation of rural properties through the performance of environmental management, marketing, finance, information technology, production and human resources activities;

b) Analysing the external and internal environment in which the company operates;

c) Present an intervention proposal to improve the performance of the rural companies analysed.

1.2 Methodology

As for the selection of participants in the study, 15 pig producers located in the municipality of São Luís in the neighbourhoods of Pedrinhas, Arraial, Quebra Pote Cidade Operaria, Tajipurú and Magril, characterised as small, medium and large producers, were surveyed.

This study used primary and secondary data. The primary data was collected through questionnaires, visits and informal conversations with employees and those responsible for the general administration of the properties. The questionnaires were made up of open and closed questions. Secondary data was obtained from documents made available by the company analysed, as well as from the Municipal Department of Agriculture, Fisheries and Supply (SEMAPA), the Brazilian Institute of Geography and Statistics (IBGE), and the

Maranhão State Agricultural Defence Agency (AGED). Once the data was available, a bibliographical survey was carried out to gain a greater theoretical understanding of the issues related to the research in question.

For a better understanding, the data was tabulated using an Excel spreadsheet and is presented in graphs for better contextualisation and understanding.

The work is structured in four chapters. The first chapter refers to the introduction. The second chapter presents the theoretical background to organisational diagnosis and the areas that make up an organisation. The third chapter presents the results of the research. The fourth chapter presents the final considerations of the work.

2 LITERATURE REVIEW

This section seeks to describe important points for a good understanding of the subject of the proposed work.

1.3 Pig farming

Pigs were domesticated in China and belong to the mammal class. The domestic pig was brought to America by Christopher Columbus and Martin Afonso de Sousa introduced the species to Brazil in 1532 (CAVALCANTI, 1985).

The world's pig herd is made up of 874.2 million animals, with China, the European Union and the United States being the biggest producers. It is estimated that data from 2013 shows that Brazil has approximately 37 million pigs, ranking fourth in the world, with the southern region of the country standing out, especially the state of Santa Catarina (IBGE, 2014). Brazil's herd has grown steadily, positively reflecting technical advances in production (ANUALPEC, 2002; IBGE, 2011). The country is also becoming an important food producer for the world, with great potential for the production and export of animal products, especially pork (ABIPECS, 2012).

Pork is the most widely produced and consumed meat in the world, along with chicken. It is therefore a food that meets consumer demands and enriches meals in a nutritious, healthy and tasty way (OLIVO; OLIVO, 2006).

In Maranhão, the herd is just over 1.2 million head, but it is the second largest producer in the Northeast, second only to the state of Bahia, but it only accounts for 4% of national production (IBGE, 2014).

According to Hadade (2011), this number will only increase due to investments, the increased production of grain in the state, which serves as animal feed, and the initiative of pig farmers, who want to create the first pig centre in Maranhão. The newspaper also states that the state will soon become a major producer of grains and animal protein and that the primary sector will become a benchmark when food exports emerge via port of Itaqui. It also mentions that the primary sector contributes more than the industrial sector and that the countryside employs 600,000 people in the state (Hadade, 2011).

1.4 Rural Administration

Rural administration is the study that deals with the organisation of an agricultural company, with a view to the efficient use of resources in order to obtain satisfactory results (BARBOSA, 1983). According to Cella (2002), this is the branch of Administration that deals with the rational processes of administrative decisions and actions in rural organisations. The author also mentions that agricultural production can be impacted by physical aspects such as: weather fluctuations, soil characteristics, water resources, availability of infrastructure and location. In addition to these, pests, crop diseases and animal diseases influence the success of farming.

Salles (1981) goes on to mention other characteristics that interfere with agricultural activity, such as the demand for productive inputs, the seasonality of the demand for credit, commercialisation problems, the perishability of some products and the irreversibility of the production process. But for Lauschner (1993), the process of commercial competition is the one that most affects agricultural activity involving both large and small producers, thus suggesting the adoption of new production strategies suited to the size of the property in order to increase competitiveness. Lauschner (1993) also presents some alternatives to reduce the disadvantages of competition in rural areas, such as: professionalisation of farming activities; integration into the agro-processing industry, as an alternative to sharing the risk; moving surplus family labour to other economic sectors; and implementing associative forms of production.

Meira (1996), when analysing agricultural activity, considered the farming environment to be "adverse to rural producers". He found that there are a large number of agricultural producers living alongside suppliers of machinery, equipment and agricultural inputs with high bargaining power and buyers of agricultural products. The rural producer also faces the threat of entry from new producers, due to the low barriers to entry and the high costs of leaving the agricultural activity, a factor that leads producers to remain in this sector even without obtaining satisfactory returns.

1.5 Organisational diagnosis

Diagnosis, also known as analysing the internal environment, is a stage in the process of analysis and planning. The dynamics of the universe of organisations justifies the continuous exercise of checking the set of variables that make up a given reality (ESCOSTEGUY; GUTFREIND, 2007). "The strategic diagnosis must focus on the current moment, as well as the next moment, the next challenge, in order to constitute the critical dimension for the permanent success of the analysed company" (OLIVEIRA, 2011, p. 64).

Organisational diagnosis is a tool that makes it possible to provide strategic information for managers to make decisions in favour of the company (ROSA, 2001). Based on the diagnosis, it is possible to identify needs and priorities and suggest effective solutions for the correct functioning of the organisation, since the systemic approach of the diagnosis is the main factor that makes it possible to achieve the objectives designed by the company's managers.

In order to carry out the organisational diagnosis, all areas of the company are analysed with the aim of discovering its weaknesses and strengths. On this occasion, adjustments will be made and new techniques suggested for better execution of the company's internal processes, with the intention of maximising the potential and development of the related areas. Through the organisational diagnosis, a new management model can be implemented, which will lead to new business behaviour.

By carrying out a business diagnosis, it will be possible to identify problems that are preventing rural property managers from achieving their objectives. In addition, diagnosing means seeking the strategic alignment of the organisation with existing resources, discovering strengths and weaknesses, the best way to take advantage of opportunities to overcome difficulties and increase the organisation's competitiveness.

The rural management model currently adopted by many small and medium-sized farms, as well as some large ones, raises concerns for various reasons. The most important of these are the management style, the lack of production cost controls, the lack of information technology, the agility of decision-making in complex situations and, especially, the lack of strategic planning. To a certain extent, these issues are generally linked to the qualification of producers to act in an organised manner in society, to control their production costs, to know the particularities of the trade in agricultural products and to manage rural property efficiently.

Business diagnostics are important for rural producers to gain an insight into the current situation of their business and its management system, as well as acquiring knowledge and experience in organisational management. In addition, they will also make a careful assessment of the property and identify its real needs, detecting management problems and organisational failures. In order to do this, they need to gather information from various sectors, getting to know the working procedures and the systemic process of the properties, in order to then draw up their restructuring plan and suggest the best decisions to be made.

In the same way as entrepreneurs in other economic activities, rural producers are also responsible for monitoring the complexity of the environment in which they operate, and are concerned with developing strategies to defend themselves against threats and take advantage of opportunities. The administrative capacity of rural producers can be considered one of the determining factors in the technical and economic results they achieve. The sequence of decisions and attitudes for conducting agricultural activities, in terms of production, finance, sales and human resources, should therefore have an impact on the performance of the rural enterprise. Organisational diagnostics is therefore a tool that helps property management, leading the producer to become a rural entrepreneur.

2.3.1 SWOT analysis: analysing strengths and weaknesses, opportunities and threats.

The management tool called SWOT analysis, which stands for Strengths, Weaknesses, Opportunities and Threats, is an instrument used for strategic planning, which makes it possible to gather information on the company's internal and external environment. SWOT analysis is also conceptualised as a "global assessment of strengths, weaknesses, opportunities and threats" (KOTLER; KELLER, 2007, p. 50). It is a tool widely used in the management of companies in urban areas, but it can and should also be used as a tool for analysing a rural company.

This tool may have been developed by an American called Albert Humphrey in research at Stanford University in the 60s and 70s. What is expected from a SWOT analysis is for the company to know its strengths in order to develop strategies to enhance them and its weaknesses in order to neutralise or avoid threats (WRIGHT, 2010).

Incidentally, SWOT analysis is one of the oldest and easiest tools to carry out. "...when properly conducted, external and internal analyses provide a wealth of information to the management team, although many of them can be confusing if examined in aggregate." (WRIGHT, 2010).

2.3.2 Internal analysis

Analysing the internal environment is what will give the company the ability to formulate its mission and objectives. As already mentioned, the company's internal analysis is represented by its strengths and weaknesses and can be considered controllable, as it is in the domain of the organisation's managers. According to Chiavenato (2000), in order to analyse a company's internal environment, various factors must be considered.

In the marketing area, the performance of the distribution system, new product development, sales force, promotion and advertising, pricing policies and the organisation of the marketing department should be diagnosed, as well as market research, which is relevant to the decision-making process.

The financial function should analyse profitability ratios, liquidity ratios, leverage ratios, turnover ratios, collection periods, planning system analysis, financial/accounting control as the structure of the financial area, cash flow reports, decisions, financial actions, controls and budgets, among others (CHIAVENATO, 2000).

In the production area, the efficiency of its production capacity is analysed, such as the industrial plant, production scheduling and control, quality, cost systems, research and development and the supply chain.

In the area of human resources, the attitudes of top management towards the company's human factor are considered, such as employee turnover, absenteeism rates, the effectiveness of recruitment, selection, training and development programmes (CHIAVENATO, 2004).

Lastly, the organisational aspects are analysed: operational and managerial information systems; the planning system (strategic, tactical and operational); the training, attitudes and behaviour of senior management and managers; the training and skills of employees; quality control; and control of the consumer market (CHIAVENATO, 2000).

2.3.3 External analysis

All companies are part of a macro environment in which they operate. Wright (2010, p. 47) confirms this by saying that "all companies are affected by political-legal, economic, technological and social trends and systems." All of these elements are present in the macro environment of organisations, so they are not within the control of the manager, as there is stability in this environment, which is complex, dynamic and limits the company's strategies.

External analysis also involves the markets covered by the company, current characteristics and future trends, opportunities, prospects and competition, i.e. companies operating in the market, competing for the same customers, consumers or resources that affect society and all other companies. Opportunities and Threats are environmental forces that are uncontrollable by the company and create obstacles to its strategic action which, for the most part, can be avoided or managed as long as they are recognised in good time (OLIVEIRA, 2011).

According to Oliveira (2011), the aim of external analysis is to study the relationship between the company and its environment in terms of opportunities and threats, as well as its current position and its future prospects. It is therefore the manager's responsibility to try to capitalise on opportunities and absorb threats or adapt to them. The macro environment in the SWOT analysis will be represented by the Opportunities and Threats quadrants. And since we have already seen that it is an unstable element, it is up to the manager to draw up strategies, creating ways for the company to function efficiently in the face of the limitations and threats imposed by the macro environment.

Oliveira (2011, p. 71) explains that the purpose of "external analysis is to study the relationship between the company and its environment in terms of opportunities and threats". This relationship, for example, could be in terms of the position of the company's product in the market. However, it is interesting that the manager tries to focus on maximising opportunities rather than reducing threats. As well as identifying which opportunities are inherent to the company's sector and which are for immediate or long-term use. Kotler and Keller (2007, p. 50) cite three main sources of market opportunities. The first is when the demand is greater than the supply, i.e. the marketing effort is much less to achieve the result. The second is to offer the consumer market the same product or service that already exists, but in a new way. There are marketing methods that help to improve an existing product, such as the problem detection method, the ideal method and the consumption chain method. The third source generally leads to a completely new product or service.

The authors also classify the opportunities in terms of Probability of Success and Attractiveness, which are shown in the four-part square, making it possible to analyse which are the best and which are the least significant opportunities. This technique can be understood by detailing each component of the SWOT tool, ensuring a better analysis in the end.

As we've seen, it's not just because the manager has spotted opportunities in the quadrant that strategies need to be put together to maximise them; we need to go beyond analysing these opportunities to decide which ones are truly relevant.

1.6 Human Resources Management

Also known as people management, it checks in practice what managers are doing to improve the productivity of people in companies. Companies that work in the People Management area usually improve the company-employee relationship, preventing future problems from arising.

Human Resources management at a strategic level allows companies to adjust to the external changes that occur in the environment in which they are inserted, moving from reactive to proactive (ALMEIDA, ET AL. 1993 p.21). The importance of the Human Resources area depends on each organisation and the valuation policy it adopts, and it can be more developed if it is considered strategic. For Chiavenato (1997, p.163), Human Resources policies depend on the philosophy and needs of each company and he also emphasises that these policies "are rules established to govern functions and ensure that they are carried out in accordance with the desired objectives".

According to the author, in order for Human Resources Management policies to be developed in a simpler way, the company needs to define the objectives that this area should achieve.

According to Chiavenato (1997, p.168) some of the objectives of Human Resources Management are:

> [...] to create, maintain and develop a contingent of human resources with the ability and motivation to achieve the organisation's objectives; to create, maintain and develop organisational conditions for the application, development and full satisfaction of human resources, and the achievement of individual objectives; and to achieve efficiency and effectiveness through the available human resources.

Once a company has defined the objectives it wants to achieve in terms of its human resources, it can adopt techniques that will make it easier to achieve these objectives.

2.4.1 Job Description and Analysis

The job description is information about: "the main tasks, duties and responsibilities involved in performing the job" (BATEMAN, 1998, p.279). Job analysis, on the other hand, is concerned with aspects related to the individual who will occupy the position. For Werther

(1983, p.107) "job analysis describes what the job requires of the employees who perform it and the human factors that are necessary." And Chiavenato (1997, p.316) says that this stage verifies the intellectual and physical qualifications needed by the occupant to perform adequately in the position.

2.4.2 Human Resources Planning

Human Resources planning is used to prepare the company to anticipate future staffing needs, avoiding staff shortages or excesses within the organisation. According to Albuquerque (1987, p.43) it is important to have Human Resources planning in order to adapt to changes in the organisation. These changes can have an impact on key issues such as: company strategies, staff demand restrictions from the external environment, administrative practices, organisational structure, management development, executive succession, long-term needs, etc. Once you have the information from your Human Resources planning and your strategic planning, the next step is to recruit to fill the planned vacancies. This is followed by training and development, human performance evaluation and remuneration.

1.7 Marketing Management

The concept of Marketing according to Gilbert & Churchill. (2012) "The process of planning and executing the conception, pricing, promotion and distribution of ideas, goods and services in order to create exchanges that satisfy individual and organisational goals", marketing can also be considered as a group of techniques and strategies used to understand and attract the attention of the public, with the aim of satisfying the customer and the company.

The first marketing model that emerged in the industrial era was called marketing 1.0, which focused exclusively on selling products on a large scale, without any interest in product quality or customer satisfaction. According to Kotler, Kartajava and Setiawan (2010, p.3) apud Reis (2020, p.11). The aim of this marketing model "was to standardise and gain in scale, in order to reduce production costs as much as possible, so that these goods could have a lower price and be acquired by a greater number of buyers".

Soon after the emergence of marketing 1.0 came marketing 2.0, which emerged in the so-called information age. Unlike marketing 2.0, marketing 2.0 focuses on customer satisfaction and the low price of the product, where everything becomes essential for customer satisfaction, while marketing 3.0 focuses on the emotions of the human being, i.e. the spirituality of the consumer.This strategy requires marketing to be more involved with the target audience because it's no longer just about selling the product as in marketing 1.0 or customer satisfaction as in marketing 2.0, it's now about understanding the consumer's needs and desires (KOTLER, KARTAJAVA & SETIAWAN, 2010, GOMES & CURY, 2013).

Marketing 4.0 is the shift from traditional to digital marketing, from physical to digital, where customers are socially connected in communications networks, in which case companies can only engage with consumers if they give them permission. According to Kotler, Kartajava and Setiawan (2017, p. 63), "Marketing 4.0 leverages machine-to-machine connectivity and artificial intelligence to improve marketing productivity, while boosting person-to-person connectivity to strengthen customer engagement".

We are currently in the era of marketing 5.0, which is marketing focussed exclusively on modern technology. This technology is beyond the capabilities of human marketers. The main objective of marketing 5.0 is to humanise and create new experiences for customers, according to Kotler, Kartajaya and Setiawan (2021, p. 19) "The technology of the future is applied to help marketers create, communicate, deliver and increase value throughout the customer journey". In today's context, digital marketing has become a trend for the hotel industry, due to the ease of access to platforms that are entirely connected to the public, such as social networks, websites and apps.

According to Kotler; Kartajaya; Setiawan (2021), segmented marketing is the method of selecting a target market divided into four segments, such as: geographical segmentation consisting of regions and localities, demographic segmentation such as age, gender, socioeconomic class, etc. Psychographic segmentation, which are selected on the basis of their beliefs, interests and motivations and finally by behavioural segmentation which determines the behaviour of consumers, such as frequent travellers, a loyal buyer, so these segments need to be connected to each other to keep the marketing relevant.

In order to carry out good marketing, you need to know the marketing strategies that are the four pillars, known as the 4 Ps of marketing or the Marketing Mix, which is an indispensable tool for planning and developing the strategies implemented in the market. According to Peçanha (2020) the 4 Ps are: Price, the amount paid for a given product or service, Product that satisfies the local consumer, Place that corresponds to the location where the product is sold, physical and virtual distribution of sales, and finally Promotion that is related to the marketing responsible for publicity, advertising, merchandising, social media, among others.

These 4 Ps must be interconnected in order to work properly and for the company's marketing to be successful in reaching its target audience of consumers. The marketing mix has existed for decades, but continues to be used and studied. It is a strategy that has not changed over the years, but has remained solid and is therefore part of the four pillars of marketing (PEÇANHA, 2020).

According to Kotler, Kartajaya and Setiawan (2017, p.25) "The flow of innovation, which used to be vertical (from companies to the market), has become horizontal." Vertical marketing is focussed exclusively on the target audience that it wants to satisfy; marketing will be aimed at the needs of this audience in order to sell the product on the market. Horizontal marketing, on the other hand, focuses on a variety of audiences, and can work with both vertical and horizontal marketing.

For Peter and Churchill (2000, p.56), marketing is the "... process of planning something or other to execute the conception of pricing, promotion and distribution of ideas, goods and services in order to create exchanges that satisfy individual and organisational goals".

In order to improve efficiency and minimise the difficulties faced by rural properties, it is necessary for rural producers to use strategies, [...] "among which value adding and product differentiation stand out" (NANTES; SCARPELLI, 2001, p.572). According to Oliveira (1991, p. 26). "adding value means raising the price of a product as a result of some change in way it is presented, whether the product *is fresh* or industrialised [...]" (ARAÚJO, 2010, p. 117).

Adding value can happen in a number of ways: "rural producers can add value to their products by classifying them according to an established standard, using suitable packaging, industrialising production and developing a brand for their product" (VILCKAS; NANTES, 2006, p. 176).

Another way of adding value to the product is through differentiation, which according to Azevedo (2000, p. 74) "[...] differentiation is a process of searching for elements that distinguish a company's product from other competing brands". Bearing in mind that small farms usually have a low scale of production, which makes it difficult to commercialise, especially products considered *commodities*, small producers should invest in producing differentiated products, such as organic, among others (NANTES; SCARPELLI, 2001).

1.8 Information Technology Management

Various factors directly affect the efficiency of a company, such as capital, technology, knowledge, the market, among others. According to Barros (2011, p. 122) "The rural environment, given its numerous activities and the financial volume of transactions (buying, selling, contracting services, production, etc.), constitutes a company, even if it is not always formally called and structured in this way." According to the author.

"A rural property is like a business, which is why decision-making should be emphasised as a factor of great importance and impact."

For Callado and Moraes Filho (2011) making the wisest decision is no easy task, as it requires knowledge of the market, anticipating trends, studying the capital involved and so on. Unfortunately, this doesn't happen in the field, as often "decisions are strictly empirical, subject to a high degree of uncertainty (NANTES; SCARPELLI, 2001, p. 563)".

Araújo (2010, p. 9) says that it is important for rural producers to have a holistic view of agribusiness, so that they can more easily monitor changes in their environment and the decision-making process becomes more precise. Among the decisions that rural producers have to make is whether or not to include new technologies. Technology is responsible for increasing productivity in the field and this is achieved through more modern machinery, new handling techniques, pesticides and fertilisers (ARAUJO, 2010). The automation of cleaning, packaging and storage processes has contributed greatly to the growth in agricultural productivity, increasing the use of available resources and maximising the capacity to generate income and foreign currency (CALLADO; CALLADO, 2011, p. 7).

However, what can be observed is that technology has not reached all rural producers due to financial issues or a lack of information and knowledge, as small producers still use rudimentary techniques that reduce the efficiency of their properties (NANTES; SCARPELLI, 2001). The intense pace of technological updating in the countryside has required the updating of information and the adoption of learning mechanisms and professional and entrepreneurial training for rural producers, which has penalised many small rural producers, who have been systematically displaced from their environment due to the need to produce in large quantities, to a high standard of quality and at competitive prices (SEGATTI; HESPANHOL, 2008, p. 616).

1.9 Environmental Management

Environmental management is a set of defined measures and procedures that, when applied correctly, reduce and control the impacts of project implementation on the environment and is standardised according to ISO (International Organisation for Standardisation) criteria. All the aspects related to the environment are described in the ISO 14,000 standards, with the management part in the ISO 14001 and 14004 standards (BARBOSA, 2007).

Environmental management is a form of administration that prioritises sustainability by using administrative practices and methods that reduce the environmental impact of economic activities on natural resources as much as possible (OLIVEIRA, 2007).

It is important for a company to adopt this type of management because it associates its image with environmental preservation and improves the image of its brands and products on the market. Organisations that adopt environmental management are able to minimise their costs, avoid waste and reuse materials that were previously discarded. They also improve their commercial relations with other companies that also follow these same principles (MAZZER & CAVALCANTI, 2004).

Nowadays, companies must have a deeper relationship with the environment in which they operate, becoming a socio-political organisation that is given responsibilities towards the environment and society (OLIVEIRA, 2007).

Changes on the world stage have led people to develop a vision of consuming products and services that are considered environmentally friendly. This vision is the result of a change in focus that is taking place in society's thinking and shifting its emphasis from the economic to the social, valuing social aspects that include fairer income distribution and quality of life (DONAIRE, 1999, p. 16).

This has forced organisations to incorporate these values into their administrative and operational procedures. Since this new market trend has shown itself to be present in society's daily life, the demand for this type of product is increasing (DONAIRE, 1999, p. 16).

Environmental problems are becoming increasingly complex and require concrete measures in relation to social, cultural, economic, political and technical factors, which are implicit in environmental impacts such as water and soil contamination that cause damage to the quality of life of living beings (BARBOSA, 2007).

In terms of environmental impacts, pig farming is classified as a productive activity with the greatest polluting potential due to the large volume of waste produced by the animals (CESCONETO; ROESLER, 2003). That's why it's very important to delve deeper into the theory of environmental quality indicators related to this rural activity, which is expanding in terms of production and technology, influenced by commercial and international competitiveness models and subject to specific environmental and inspection standards, which are increasingly consolidating corrective measures and alternatives for adapting pig farming activities based on viable and real proposals for managing environmental assets (ROESLER, 2002).

1.10Financial Management

Financial planning helps solve problems and make decisions. Knowledge of finance helps rural entrepreneurs to perform their duties well (CREPALDI, 2011). In addition, the rural entrepreneur or manager needs to know accounting and finance in order to understand the financial reports prepared by the organisation. Finance provides a means of liaison that facilitates communication between the different departments and also provides indications of how each department can conduct its activities (CREPALDI, 2011).

The manager of an enterprise needs to know where and how he is investing his resources and what the financial return is by classifying and organising the data relating to the daily economic and financial movement of the property (CREPALDI, 2011). This is because managers need to know how profitable their production activity is, what results have been obtained and how they can be optimised by evaluating results, sources of income and types of expenditure and how to improve income and reduce expenditure.

3 RESULTS AND DISCUSSION

A discussion of the results of the research involving the functional diagnosis of rural property areas is presented. It should be emphasised that one of the aims of strategic diagnosis is to provide information so that management has maximum knowledge of the company's environment. To achieve this, it is necessary to carry out a detailed analysis of the organisation and its environment.

With regard to the categories of analysis, these are classified as internal environments, comprising the strengths and weaknesses of the companies analysed, and external environments, delimited by the opportunities and threats faced by these companies.

In order to facilitate the organisation of the data and the understanding of the results, the option was made to present the data in the form of topics.

1.11 Production and Operations

The data shows that the production capacity of 60% of the properties ranged from 15 to 400 head of pigs and that 40% of them ranged from 1,500 to 5,800 head of pigs, but none of them used the facilities in their entirety. This can be explained by the lack of own resources on most of the properties and the planning of farrowings on the property with the largest number of animals.

Of the properties analysed, 93.3% carry out other activities, such as raising fish, free-range poultry, cassava and vegetables, and only 6.7% of them had pig farming as their only activity.

As for controlling production costs, 86.7 per cent don't do it at all, 13.3 per cent write down their costs and revenues in a notebook and only one uses computers with appropriate software.

Stocks of medicines and food are present on 86.7 per cent of farms and 13.3 per cent don't stock anything.

In 93.3 per cent of the properties the facilities and equipment are in good condition, but in 6.7 per cent of them the facilities are in poor condition.

Of the producers surveyed, 66.7 per cent said that they receive technical assistance sporadically, while 33.3 per cent do not receive any at all and, consequently, 93.3 per cent of farms do not make innovations in the production process due to a lack of guidance.

Some of this information can be seen in Figure 1.

Figure 1 - Production capacity, facility conditions, cost control, input stocks and technical assistance.

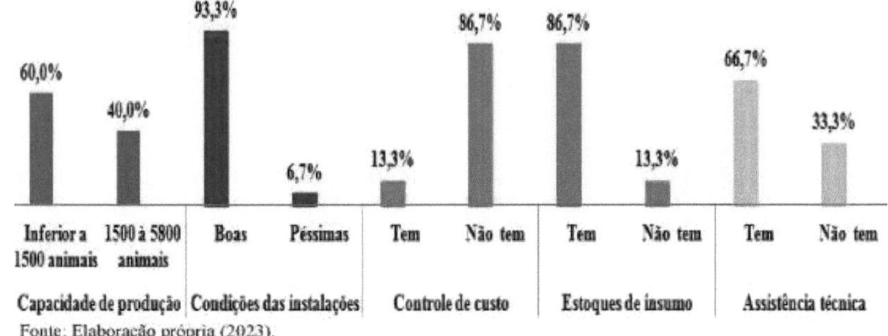

Fonte: Elaboração própria (2023).

1.12 Commercialisation and Marketing

The results showed that 66.7% of farms sell live animals, while 33.3% sell them live and/or slaughtered. Of the total analysed, 86.7% sell to supermarkets, market stalls, butchers, restaurants and other producers, while only 13.3% sell directly to the end consumer at the door. As for where they sell, 66.7% sell only in the neighbourhood where they live and 33.3% manage to sell to several neighbourhoods in the city. 93.3% of the owners said that their products are well accepted in the market and that they manage to sell everything they produce, so much so that sometimes they can't meet demand. This is due to the fact that the pork market in Brazil has grown steadily, and this product is now a bigger part of Brazilians' diets.

However, 73.3% do not have records with health inspection bodies and only 27.7% said they were registered with the Maranhão Agricultural Defence Agency (AGED). This lack of sanitary control in a way ends up limiting the consumption of pork by the more conscientious ludovicenses, since consumers are increasingly concerned about obtaining food with acceptable hygienic and sanitary quality in accordance with inspection standards.

Of the farms surveyed, 90.9% don't advertise their product in any way. Only 9.1% use the media to publicise their product, such as television, billboards and buses. When asked if they did any market research, 86.7% replied that they don't do any research and 13.3% do some kind of research, such as getting to know their competitors and suppliers It became very clear during the survey that the majority of producers don't include a market vision in their day-to-day business.

However, farms in general have been achieving good market results. This is partly due to the average trading prices of the animals, as the price of a live piglet varies from R$120.00 to R$150.00, while the cuts vary from R$8.00 to R$12.00 depending on the neighbourhood where they are produced. Another factor that guarantees the competitiveness of the breeders is the quality and good levels of weight gain of the animals due to the use of breeds that are highly precocious, which allows the properties to achieve good performances in the negotiations.

Some of this information can be seen in Figure 2.

Figure 2 - Forms of sale, place of sale, buyers and product promotion.

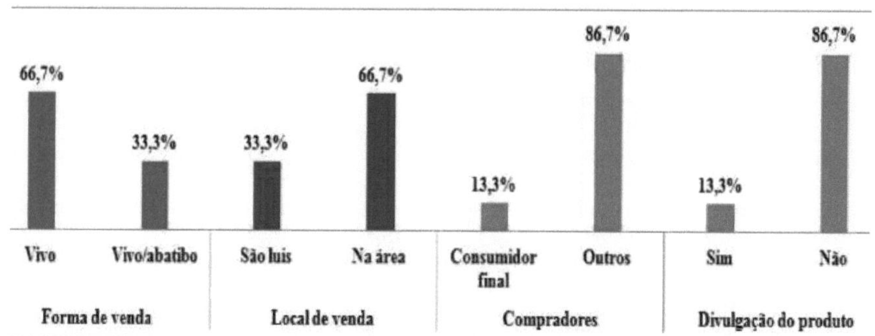

Source: Own elaboration (2023).

1.13Management Information System

Figure 3 shows that 93.3 per cent of producers have no or only one employee and that only one company has more than one employee (6.7 per cent).

Figure 3 - Number of employees, family support, computer use.

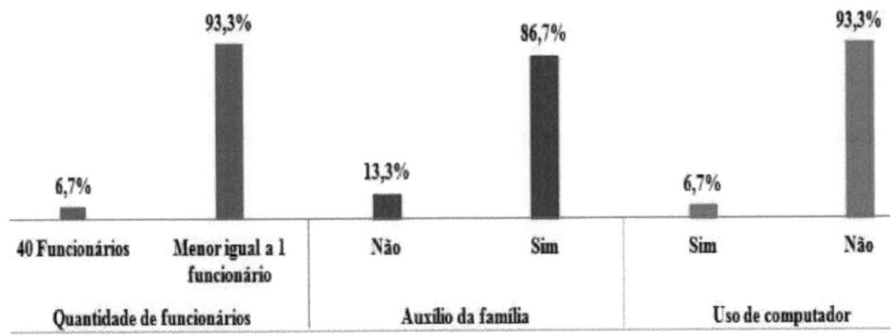

Fonte: Elaboração própria (2023).

As for the presence of a computer, 93.3% of the producers said that they didn't have one or that they had one but didn't use it because they didn't know how to use computers. Only 6.7% use this equipment (one company). As for labour, 86.7% are helped directly by their families and 13.3% say they work alone.

It is clear from the research that, despite living in the information age, it is still a reality that the majority of producers do not use information technology, as the research reflects their lack not only financially, but also of knowledge of this tool, which is fundamental for generating more reliable information on the productive performance of the activity and helping to make the necessary decisions in relation to the activity.

3.4 Administrative Management

As shown in Figure 4, the administrative management of the farms analysed has as its main points of relevance the reason that led the producers to undertake this activity. Of the total, 66.7% said it was due to family tradition and 33.3% said it was by chance, influence from other farmers, bank projects and even passion. When asked, all of them said they thought they were experienced in the business, but 86.7% said they were committed to their property's growth objectives.

However, sustainable growth is only possible if the objectives are defined based on the commitment of the people involved in the activities as a whole, making it easier to coordinate efforts, as only 6.7% of them work as a team, even when it comes to their own family labour. Of all the producers surveyed, 93.3% say that they alone make decisions on the farm, such as negotiating prices.

Despite having considerable experience in the activity, the management of the owners is considered rigid, which is a negative point for the property, as this rigidity could affect the performance of the workers and the family labour force itself in terms of the planned results. In this case, the property's performance can suffer, as some problems that could be resolved quickly can become major barriers to the development of productive activities due to the concentration and rigidity of decisions.

Figure 4 - Reason for joining the business, decision-making power and commitment to objectives.

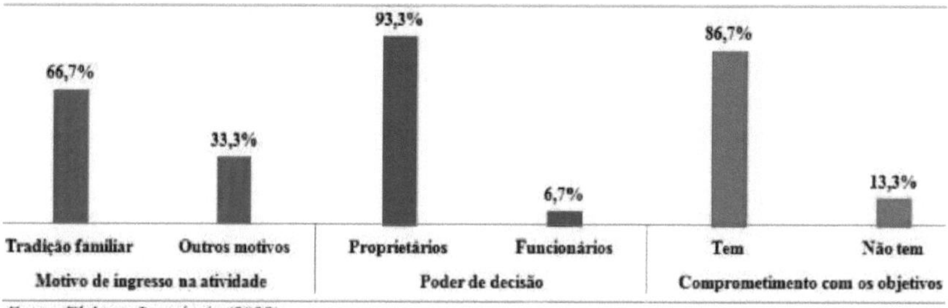

66,7%
33,3%
93,3%
6,7%
86,7%
13,3%
Tradição familiar
Outros motivos
Motivo de ingresso na atividade
Proprietários
Funcionários
Poder de decisão
Tem
Não tem
Comprometimento com os objetivos

Fonte: Elaboração própria (2023).

One positive point that stood out was the fact that all the producers showed some kind of understanding of the activity involved in pig farming. What's more, the answers indicate that they have learning potential and experience in this area of knowledge, even if it's incipient.

3.5 Financial Management

Figure 5 shows the financial management of the farms analysed. 86.7% of the producers said that they manage to honour their commitments with the income generated by their production, but 93.3% do not have any capital reserves for any problems or investments. Of the producers surveyed, 20% have PRONAF credit or other bank credit, such as personal credit, which they invest in the property, but 80% of them do not have any type of credit, so they say they do not have any debts.

Figure 5 - Profitable activity, income to pay commitments, debts, accounting.

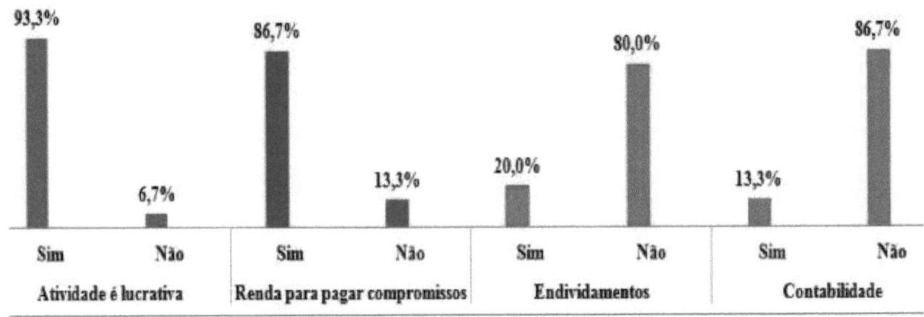

Fonte: Elaboração própria (2023).

When asked about the profitability of the activity, 93.3% said that it was profitable. However, the lack of transparent financial statements prevents producers from having concrete information about the current profitability situation and at the same time prevents them from using important investment risk management tools, such as viability indicators, net present value and internal rate of return, because 86.7% of the producers surveyed don't keep accounts to confirm their profitability and 13.3% make notes in specific programmes or in a notebook about the sales and expenses generated in the activity. 93.3% don't pay any kind of tax and 93.3% don't even calculate equipment depreciation. However, 100% of producers maintain their facilities.

There is no doubt that money is one of the main means of stimulating an individual or group of workers to mobilise to improve their quality of life. However, if the worker doesn't have good management skills or technical assistance to manage the financial resources, it turns from a positive reinforcer into a negative one, with drastic consequences for the personal and social lives of these workers, as in the case of the producers who had debts.

3.6 Human Resources Management

The Human Resources Area is considered to exist in only one property (6.7% of the total analysed), where specialised labour was found, with employee selection, contractual formalisation, low staff turnover, motivation and qualification (Figure 6). In the others, family labour was used to a large extent, without neglecting the appearance of other forms of participation, such as just the action of the producer or a single employee.

As for professional qualifications, 53.3 per cent of the producers surveyed have already taken part in courses or lectures, but 46.7 per cent have never done any kind of qualification.

Figure 6 - Qualification activity and skilled labour.

93,3%
53,3%
46,7%
6,7%
Sim
Não
Sim
Não
Atividade de qualificação
Mão de obra especializada

3.7 Environmental Management

Figure 7 shows the area of environmental management, more specifically the procedures carried out by the farms regarding the destination of their waste. In 53.3% of the farms, the waste is dried in the sun and used to fertilise plants, while in 46.7% it goes into pits (boxes for decomposition) and settling ponds, without a final destination. One of the companies surveyed is planning to set up biodigesters. As for cleaning the facilities, 33.3 per cent do it dry, while 73.3 per cent use water. In 86.7 per cent of the properties the drinking fountains are of the dummy type and in 13.3 per cent plastic containers are placed on the ground.

Figure 7 - Cleaning, waste disposal, types of drinking troughs.

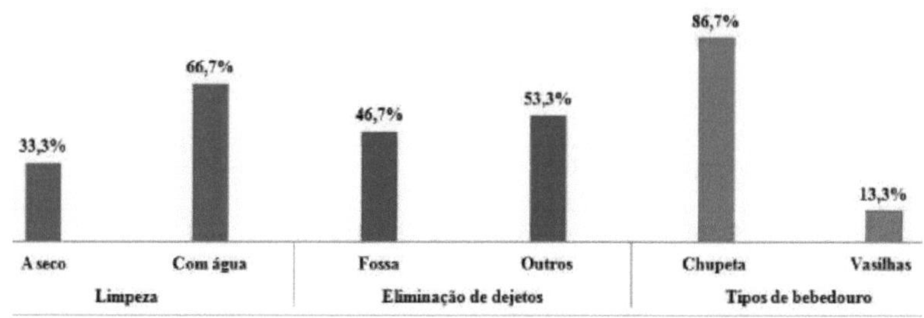

Source: Own elaboration (2023).

3.8 Analysing the internal and external environment of pig farms

To carry out this analysis, we used the framework constructed from the SWOT analysis. Among the strengths identified on the farms, the production is easy to commercialise, as none of the producers reported problems with sales. Another important strength is the use of local businesses. Lastly, the strong point identified was the location, where access is easy (Chart 1). As can be seen from the data collected in the questionnaires, the weak point cited was the lack of technical assistance, which is very important for the development of production, as well as the lack of labour, which some producers complain they can't find in the area where they are located. The lack of water in some of the communities where some of the producers are located and the lack of control over production costs are also weak points.

Table 1 - SWOT analysis of the farms analysed

SWOT analysis		
	S. Forces	**W. Weaknesses**
INTERNAL ENVIRONMENT	1. Easy-to-market production; 2. Facilities in good condition; 3. Good location (areas within 20 kilometres of trade fairs or commercial points); 4. Competitive prices; 5. Utilisation of local businesses; 6. Input stocks.	1. Lack of sales strategies; 2. Lack of control over production costs; 3. Lack of labour; 4. Lack of water in some properties; 5. Lack of technical assistance.
	O. Opportunities	**T. Threats**
EXTERNAL ENVIRONMENT	1. Significant increase in consumer income; 2. Demographic development; 3. Market acceptance of the product;	1. Facilities for new entrants; 2. Distance from food suppliers; 3. Lack of government incentives; 4. High food prices;

	4. Expansion capacity;	5. Difficulties in acquiring food.
	5. Growing demand for your products	6. Lack of health inspections

Source: Own elaboration adapted from Kotler Keller (2007).

With regard to opportunities, the data collected revealed that the products are well accepted in the market, which is related to the good quality combined with the growing demand for agricultural products. The ability to expand is a significant opportunity that rural property has to exploit, as well as technology at the service of productivity, which generates a drop in operating costs and greater productivity.

With regard to the threats faced by the farms, we highlight the difficulty in acquiring food, since practically all the farms buy from CONABE and CONABE doesn't always have this food available at the time requested by the producers, so they turn to local businesses or buy from other cities, as is the case with soya, which they buy from Balsas. In addition to the distance from suppliers, the high prices of food and the lack of government incentives end up seriously affecting the competitiveness of pig farming in São Luis.

4 BUSINESS INTERVENTION PROPOSAL

At this stage, after the organisational diagnosis, proposals for improvements are presented. The aim is to get producers to develop mechanisms that allow them to grow through the opportunities found in analysing the external environment.

On the other hand, it is suggested that control mechanisms be put in place so that the owner can monitor this growth and make decisions to increase productivity in the short and long term.

The proposals were made on the basis of the internal and external environments presented in Table 1, based on the tool presented in the SWOT analysis. The idea was to come up with simple and objective proposals for improvement, at little or no cost, bearing in mind the reality of rural properties. In this way, the aim is to achieve the willingness of producers and employees to accept and implement the changes proposed in this work.

The proposals for producers/properties are described below:

a) Seek registration of the activity with the relevant bodies;

b) Keep track of the costs and income from the activity(ies). This is important to see if the activity is profitable or not and where you can cut costs. For those producers who have more than one activity, it also serves to see which activity can be discarded, thus freeing up (very scarce) financial resources and labour for more profitable activities;

c) Utilising as much of their productive capacity as possible through better planning of calving on the farm;

d) Professional training for producers and employees/family members through courses on business management, pig farming, the importance of the market in agricultural activity, health regulations, etc. Especially for those producers who have never taken part in any training;

e) Strengthen existing associations and try to get technical assistance through them;

f) Through the associations, they seek to create their own brand for the product, reducing competition, increasing production quality and increasing competitiveness;

g) Add value to the product by slaughtering the animals and selling directly to the consumer. It could strengthen existing local businesses or expand to other neighbourhoods, taking advantage of the growing demand for pork and the growing population of São Luís;

h) Producers should seek out the opinions of family members or employees who are closest to customers in order to work together, so that the organisation can gather the strength it needs to tackle its weaknesses;

i) Finally, even if the produce is easy to sell, as the producers said, there is a need for publicity and advertising with a view to future production, so this should be intensified in the neighbourhood where the farms are located. Even though word-of-mouth marketing already exists, which by the way is the cheapest and most efficient, simple models can be sought, such as the use of cars and bicycles with sound systems and information leaflets.

5 FINAL CONSIDERATIONS

The literature review carried out for this work makes clear the complexity of the organisational diagnosis of a company, but it is also even clearer that it is impossible to find all of its components in a rural company, particularly one that raises pigs like those found in São Luís, most of which are small and medium-sized properties and are family-run. However, due to its importance, it shouldn't be discarded even for these properties, because in order for a business to thrive, it needs to provide sufficient economic results to cover all expenses, remunerate the owner and generate a profit so that the necessary investments can be made, even if they are small, and, furthermore, the constant adaptation of the activity to changes in the economic reality and in consumer taste and preference, is mainly the responsibility of small producers as a matter of economic survival and social reproduction.

The market has evolved a great deal, both economically and socially and culturally, causing organisations at all levels to look for strategies to become competitive and remain in the emerging market. Researching a model that meets the diverse situations found in the rural world is no longer as difficult as it was in years gone by. Today we have an arsenal of models that can help with the business management of any rural company.

After discussing the results of the research, it can be said that the environmental diagnosis of rural properties specialising in pig production is fundamental for supporting decisions on the construction of actions aimed at developing a strategic management plan, as well as providing important information for action by professionals and local public bodies.

According to what has been reported throughout the work, it can be seen that the perspectives involved in the management of properties specialising in pig breeding are embedded in a complexity of processes and operations that imposes a delimitation on expectations regarding organisational objectives, so the analysis of external and internal variables, carried out using the *SWOT* analysis model, is fundamental for effective decision-making on strategic actions and initiatives in the development of production and marketing activities. Its simplicity and efficiency are also noteworthy.

However, after collecting the data and information on the behaviour of the internal environment variables, it allowed for a greater understanding of the functionality of the current administrative system of the farms, as well as indicating the performance of the activity in relation to the environment in which they operate. However, analysing the results of the micro-environment provides a representative discussion of the activities carried out by the farms, significantly broadening their planning horizon.

This does not end the countless possibilities for further work on this subject, as the world's population increases and the need for food follows suit. Therefore, may this work be a source of up-to-date data on the subject and may it guide the realisation of others with the generation of knowledge and techniques capable of improving the efficiency and results of agricultural economic activities, in particular pig farming in São Luís.

REFERENCES

ABIPECS. **Brazilian Association of Pork Producers and Exporters. 2012.** Available at: <http://www.abpecs.org.br>. Accessed on 28 November 2014.

ALBUQUERQUE, L. G. **Strategic role of human resources**. 1987. 262 f. (Honours thesis) - Faculty of Economics, Administration and Accounting,

University of São Paulo. São Paulo, 1987.

ALMEIDA, Martinho Isnard Ribeiro de et al. Why Strategically Manage Human Resources? **Revista de Administração de Empresas**, São Paulo: AESP/FGV, 1993.

ANUALPEC. **Yearbook of Brazilian Agronomy. São Paulo:** Fonseca, São Paulo, 2002. 284 p.

ARAÚJO, M. J. **Fundamentos de agronegócios.** 3. ed. São Paulo: Atlas, 2010.

AZEVEDO, P. F. Competition in agribusiness. In: ZYLBERSZTAJN, D.; NEVES, M. F. **Economics and management of agri-food businesses**. São Paulo: Pioneira, 2000. p. 61-79.

BALLANTYNE, David. - A relationship-mediated theory of internal marketing. "European Journal of Marketing, 2003, Vol.37, No.9, p.1242-1260.

BARBOSA, J. S. **Administração rural em nível de fazendeiro**. São Paulo, Nobel, 1983.

BARBOSA, F. A. **Administration of cattle farms**. Viçosa: Aprenda fácil, 2007.

BARROS, I. O. Auditing in rural companies. In: CALLADO, A. A. C. **Agronegócio**. 3. ed. São Paulo: Atlas, 2011. p. 120-132.

BATEMAN, Thomas S. **Administração**: construindo vantagem competitiva. São Paulo: Atlas, 1998.

CALLADO, A. A. C.; CALLADO, A. L. C. C. Agro-industrial systems. In: CALLADO, A. A. C. **Agronegócio**. 3. ed. São Paulo: Atlas, 2011. p. 1-19.

CALLADO, A. A. C.; MORAES FILHO, R. A. Business management in agribusiness. In: CALLADO, A. A. C. **Agronegócio**. 3. ed. São Paulo: Atlas, 2011. p. 20-29.

CAVALCANTI, S. de S. **Produção de suínos**. 2. ed. Campinas: Instituto Campeiro de

Ensino Agrícola, 1985.

CELLA, D. **Characterisation of the factors related to the success of a rural entrepreneur**. 2002. 166p. Dissertation (Master's in Applied Economics) - Luiz de Queiroz College of Agriculture, University of São Paulo. Piracicaba, 2002.

CESCONETO, E. A; ROESLER, M. R. B. **Partial report of the training course for technicians**: environmental management in pig farming. Toledo: UNIOESTE, 2003.

CHIAVENATO, Idalberto. **Administration**: theory, process and practice. 4 ed. Rio de Janeiro: Elsevier, 2007. 309 p.

. **Human resources**, 4. ed. São Paulo: Atlas, 1997.

. **Introduction to general management theory**: 2. ed. Rio de Janeiro: Campus, 2000.

. **The new paradigms**. 5. ed. São Paulo: Manole, 2010.

. **Administração nos novos tempos.** 2. ed. Rio de Janeiro: Elseiver, 2004.

CHIAVENATO, Idalberto; NETO, E. P. C. **Strategic management**. São Paulo: Saraiva 2003

CREPALDI, S. A. **Rural accounting**: a decision-making approach. 6.ed. São Paulo: Atlas, 2011.

DONAIRE, Denis. Environmental Management in the Company. 2.ed. São Paulo: Atlas, 1999.

ESCOSTEGUY, Ana Carolina D.; GUTFREIND, Cristiane Freitas (eds.). **Readings in communication, culture and technology.** Porto Alegre: Edipucrs, 2007.

HADADE, Lucas. **Maranhão is the second largest pork and beef producer in the Northeast**.

2011. Available at:

<http://www.oimparcial.com.br/app/noticia/negocios/2011/07/01/intema_negocios,85392/maranhao-e-o-segundo-produtor-de-carne-suina-e-bovina-do-nordeste.shtml >. Accessed on 03 no. 2014.

IBGE. Brazilian Institute of Geography and Statistics. **IBGE indicators.** 2011.

Available at: < http://www.ibge.gov.br >. Accessed on 08 October 2014.

. **Municipal Livestock Survey**. 2014. Available at: <http://www.sidra.ibge.gov.br/bda/tabela/protabl.asp?c=3939&z=t&o=24&i=P>. Accessed 10 Nov. 2014.

KOTLER, Philip; KELLER, Kevin Lane. **Marketing management**: the **marketing** bible. 12. ed. São Paulo: Pearson, 2007. 56 p.

KOTLER, P., & KELLER, K. L. (2012). **Marketing management.** São Paulo: Pearson Prentice Hall.

KOTHER, Philip; KARTAJA YA, Hermawan; SETIAWAN, Iwan. **Marketing 4.0 from traditional to digital**. Rio de Janeiro: Gmt Editora Ltda, 2017.

KOTLER, Philip; KARTAJAYA, Hermawan; SETIAWAN, Iwan. **Marketing 5.0 technology for humanity**. Rio de Janeiro: Sextante, 2021.

LAUSCHNER, R. **Agribusiness, co-operatives and rural producers**. São Leopoldo: Unisinos, 1993. 293 p.

MAZZER , Cassiano;CAVALCANTI,Osvaldo Albuquerque. Introduction to environmental waste management. Infarma, v.16, p.12-16, 2004.

MEIRA, J. L. **Economic success and the entrepreneurial strategist profile of rural producers**: the Nilo Coelho case. Lavras, 1996, 76 p. (Master's dissertation) - School of Agriculture, Federal University of Lavras. Lavras, 1996.

NANTES, J. F. D.; SCARPELLI, M. Production management in agribusiness. In: BATALHA, M. O. **Gestão agroindustrial**. 2. ed. Vol. 1. São Paulo: Atlas, 2001. p. 556-584.

OLIVEIRA, Flavio. Eco-efficiency: environmental value management São Paulo: ESPE, 2007.

OLIVEIRA, Djalma de Pinho Rebouças de. **Planejamento Estratégico**: conceitos, metodologia e práticas. 29. ed. São Paulo: Atlas, 2011.

OLIVEIRA, D. P. R. **Business strategy**: an entrepreneurial approach. 2.ed. São Paulo: Atlas,

1991.

OLIVO, R; OLIVO, N. Production and market. In: **The world of meat:** science, technology & market. P.139-149. Criciúma, 2006.

PAPASOLOMOU-DOUKAKIS, Loanna - Internal Marketing in the UK Retail Banking Sector: Rhetoric or Reality? "**Journal of Marketing Management**", 2003, 19, p.197-224.

PEÇANHA, Vitor. **4 Ps of Marketing: understand everything about the Marketing Mix concept**. 2020. Available at: https://rockcontent.com/br/blog/4-ps-do-marketing/ . Accessed on: 14 June 2023.

PETER, J. Paul; CHURCHILL, Girbert. **Marketing creating value for your customers.** 2nd ed. São Paulo: Saraiva, 2000.

REIS, Tiago. **Back office: what is it? How important is this area in a company?** 2021. Available at: https://www.suno.com.br/artigos/back-office/ . Accessed on: 16 June 2023.

ROESLER, M. R. B; CESCONETO, E. A. **Study of environmental indicators**: concepts and applications in environmental management projects in the Paraná III Basin. Toledo: UNIOESTE, 2002 (Report: Actions of the National Environment Programme II (PNMA II) and Cultivating Good Water).

ROSA, José Antônio. **Roteiro para análise e diagnóstico da empresa**. São Paulo: STS, 2001.

SALLES, S. B. **Effects of a system of agricultural registers on the managerial efficiency of rural entrepreneurs**: the case of the Fidene system in Rio Grande do Sul. 1981. 98p. (Master's dissertation) - Faculty of Economic Sciences, Federal University of Rio Grande do Sul. Porto Alegre, 1981.

SEGATTI, S.; HESPANHOL, A. N. **Alternatives for generating income on small rural properties.** 2008. Available at: < http://w3.ufsm.br/gpet/engrup/ivengrup/pdf/segatti_e_hespanhol.pdf >. Accessed on: 07 July 2014.

VILCKAS, M.; NANTES, J. F. D. Planning and adding value in rural enterprises. In: ZUIN,

L. F. S.; QUEIROZ, T. R. **Agronegócios:** Gestão e inovação. 3. ed. São Paulo: Saraiva, 2006. p. 167-188.

WERTHER, William B. **Personnel management and human resources**. São Paulo: McGraw-Hill, 1983.

WRIGHT, Peter. et al. **Strategic Management**: Concepts. 1. ed. São Paulo: Atlas, 2010.

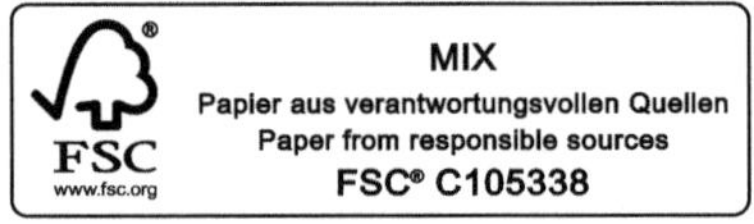

Printed by Books on Demand GmbH, Norderstedt / Germany